The An low carb food list

A beginner's guide on real food to eat without getting fat.

Plus eat to lose weight

Beatrice .K. MacBrown

Copyright

All Rights Reserved. Contents in this book may not be copied in any way or by means without the written consent of the publisher, with the exclusion of brief excerpt in critical reviews and articles.

Beatrice .K. MacBrown© 2020

Disclaimer

This book is projected to be a general guide, to raise consciousness, and to aid people to make knowledgeable decisions in the context of their circumstance.

The author takes no responsibility for any damage or injury be it personal or monetary, as a result of the use or abuse of the information in this book. If you have any doubts or worries after reading this book, do well to speak to a qualified person before further actions.

Table of content

Chapter One 5

  Introduction 5

Chapter Two 8

  Egg and Meat 8

    List of egg and meat 8

Chapter Three 14

  Seafood 14

    List of Seafood 14

Chapter Four 18

  Shell food 18

    List of shell food 18

Chapter Five 21

  Vegetables 21

    List of Vegetables 21

Chapter Six 33

  Fruits and berries 33

    Lists of fruits and berries 33

Chapter Seven 40

Nuts and seeds	40
Lists of Nuts and Seeds	40
Chapter Eight	49
Dairy	49
List of dairy	49
Chapter Nine	54
Fats and Oils	54
Lists of fats and oils	54
Chapter Ten	56
Beverages	56
Other Food	57

Chapter One

Introduction

Low carb is any diet lower than 130 grams of carbs per day. Low carb is a flexible way of eating that permits you to choose carbohydrates level that works for your health and lifestyle. Consuming fewer carbs in your meal is more effective for weight loss without going hungry, and also lower sugar level, or for reversing type 2 diabetes. Eating fewer carbs can also be more challenging.

It would be best if you chose a level of carbohydrate that is good for your system.

Below are researched carbohydrates intakes per day:

Moderate carbohydrate: 130 to 225g of carbs

Low carbohydrate: under 130g of carbs

Very-low carbohydrate: under 30g of carbs

What does a low carb diet do? A low-carb diet reduces carbohydrates and highlights more on foods high in fat and protein. There are a lot of low carb diets existing in our world today. Each diet comes with its restrictions on the types and quantity of carbohydrates you can consume.

The aim of a low-carb diet is for weight loss, and at times, it attracts many health benefits such as reducing the risk factors that come with metabolic syndrome.

The magic behind consuming low carb diet is that it decreases carbs and lowers insulin levels; this metabolism causes the body to burn stockpiled fat for energy, thereby leading to weight loss.

Low carb is when you restrict the amount and type of carbohydrates you eat. Carbohydrates are a type of calorie giving macronutrient present in various foods and beverages. Common examples of such foods that naturally contain carbohydrates: Grains, Fruits, Vegetables, Milk, Nuts, and Seeds, Legumes (beans, lentils, and peas). Some foods that contain refined carbohydrates are: white loaves of bread, pasta, cake, cookies, candy, drinks and sugar-sweetened soda. Drastically cut in carb can lead to many temporary health effects in some individuals, such as Headache, Bad breath, Weakness, Muscle cramps, Fatigue, Skin rash, Constipation, or diarrhea.

Low carb diets are not for preteens and high schoolers because their growing bodies require the nutrients in whole grains of vegetables and fruits.

Inform your doctor before you start any weight-loss diet, particularly if you have any health challenges, such as heart disease or diabetes.

Below are the 100 amazing low carb diet lists with their percentage.

For easy evaluation, all numbers are grams of digestible carbs per 100 grams (3½ ounces) serving.

Chapter Two

Egg and Meat

List of egg and meat

1. **Eggs (almost zero)**

An egg is one of the most nourishing and healthiest known foods on earth.

It contains low Carb.

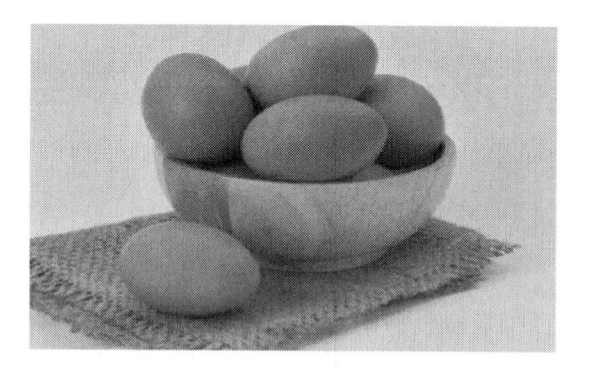

Benefits

- One large boiled egg contains a little bit of every nutrient you need

Eggs contain moderate amounts of vitamin D, vitamin B6, vitamin E, vitamin K, calcium, and zinc.

- Eggs contain a high amount of cholesterol but do not harmfully affect cholesterol in the blood when consumed. the
- It raises the "good" cholesterol in the body known as HDL (high-density lipoprotein).
- It contains Choline which helps in building cell membranes and plays a role in producing signaling molecules in the brain
- When an egg is consumed, it appears to change the form of LDL particles from small, dense LDL (bad) to large LDL. Large LDL is linked to a lower heart disease risk.
- Eggs contain powerful antioxidants Lutein and Zeaxanthin, which reduce the risk of cataracts and macular degeneration.
- Omega-3 enriched and pastured eggs may contain high amounts of omega-3 fatty acids, which help to lower blood triglycerides.
- Eggs are high in Quality Protein, which is the primary building block in the human body.
- According to many studies, Egg DOES NOT increases the risk of Heart disease and may lower the risk of stroke.
- Eggs are incredibly filling, highly satisfying, and, it also promotes weight loss.

- Eggs are nature perfect food, and eating up to three whole eggs per day is perfectly okay according to studies.

2. Beef (Zero)

Beef is highly satisfying and loaded with vital nutrients that you need to survive.

It contains zero CARB, iron, and vitamin B12, B3 and B6, selenium, and zinc.

The beef comes in different types from ribeye steak to hamburger to ground beef, and the nutrients vary depending on the food intake.

You are what you eat; the food cow eats affects the nutrient composition of its beef, especially in the area of fatty acid composition.

Grass-fed beef contains less fat and calories when compared to grain-fed beef.

Grass-fed beef is high in CLA, omega-3 fatty acids, and vitamin E, which are beneficial to health.

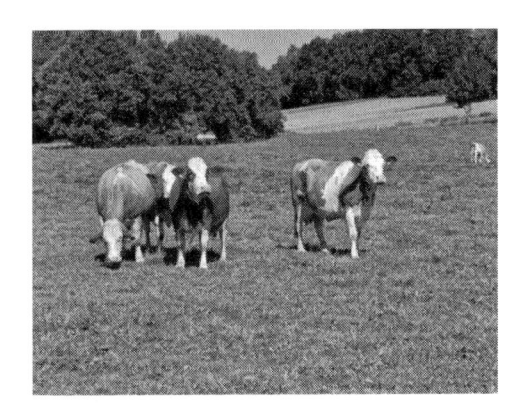

3. Lamb (Zero)

Lamb is loaded with beneficial nutrients.

It contains ZERO CARB, iron, and vitamin B12.

Lamb is mainly grass-fed and high in the beneficial fatty acid conjugated linoleic acids.

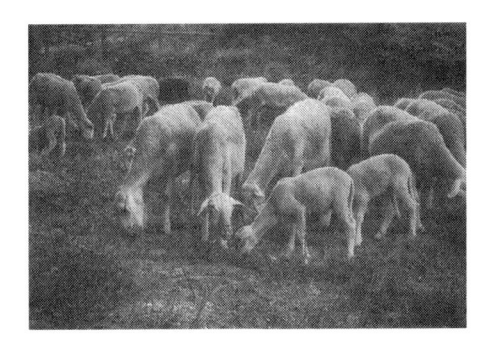

CLA present in grass-fed lamb can help improve body composition by lowering body fat levels and increases muscle mass.

4. Chicken

Chicken is a delicious meat that is widely consumed and also good source of protein.

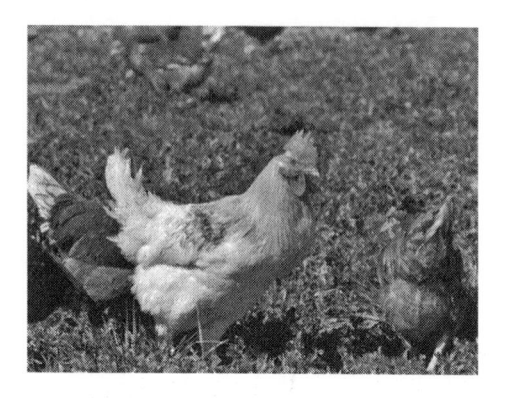

It contains ZERO CARB and is high in many beneficial nutrients

Chicken wings and thighs are an excellent choice for those on a low carb diet.

Chicken (breast) is ideal meat for fitness enthusiasts because it helps them reach their health and fitness goals by building and maintaining muscle.

If you want to lose weight, try to eat chicken breast, it has fewer calories when compared to other parts of the chicken.

5. Pork / Bacon

Pork is delicious and highly nutritious meat.

Bacon is processed meat (pork), and it acceptable to be consumed on a moderate amount. Many people on the low-carb diet enjoy eating bacon. If you must eat bacon, try to buy it locally without artificial ingredients, avoid the one that is cured with sugar.

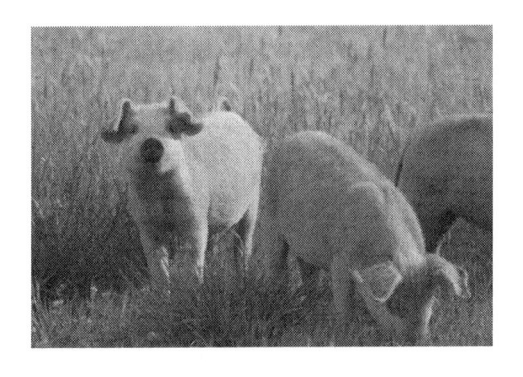

Bacon is all about fat; it contains about 50% monounsaturated fat with oleic acid taking more significant percentage, 40% saturated fat and 10 % polyunsaturated fat

The saturated fat and cholesterol in bacon are not as harmful as portrayed according to the study. Bacon is best when consumed in small quantities. Bacon is a good source of vitamins and minerals

NOTE:

Avoid eating a lot of pork because of its high salt content; it increases blood pressure in salt-sensitive people.

Chapter Three

Seafood

List of Seafood

Seafood is exceptional, incredibly in nutrition, and health.

They're high in B12, iodine and omega-3 fatty acids

1. Salmon

It contains ZERO CARB

Salmon is tasty and highly nutritious food, most popular among health-conscious individuals. It possesses a unique, delicate flavor with little or no fishy taste.

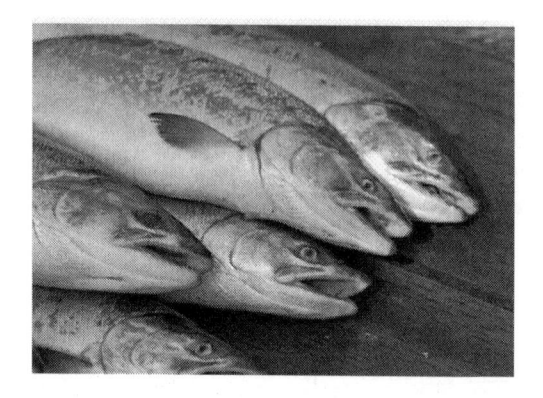

- It contains long-chain omega-3 fatty acids, Vitamins B12, iodine, and a moderate amount of vitamins D3.
- It is rich in high-quality protein.
- Salmon fish is a good source of B vitamins.

- Salmon is rich in potassium.
- It is rich in selenium
- It contains the antioxidant astaxanthin, which gives the fish its red pigment.
- It lowers the risk of heart disease
- When frequently consumed it helps in weight loss and maintenance.

2. **Trout**

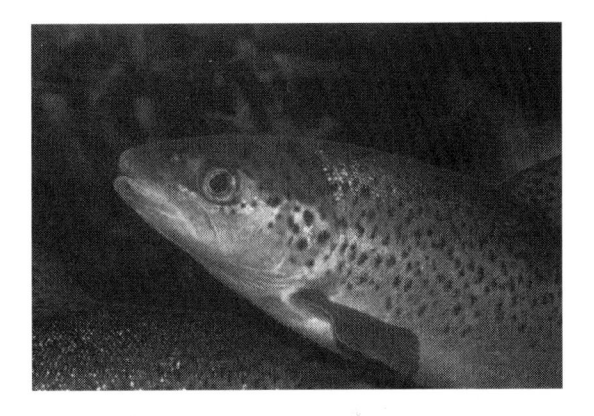

It also classified as a fatty fish that is high in long-chain omega-3 fatty acids and many vital nutrients.

It has ZERO CARB

3. **Sardines**

Sardines contain virtually every single nutrient needed in the body. It can be eaten with the bone inclusive. It is an oily fish loaded with essential nutrients and most sought for in the world.

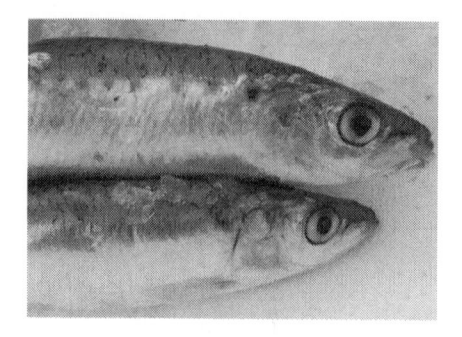

It contains ZERO CARB and abundant in magnesium, selenium, potassium, and B vitamins.

4. Tuna

Tuna is a healthy food with high nutritional value.

It contains ZERO CARB, no fiber

Tuna provides the body with minerals, vitamins and other food nutrients

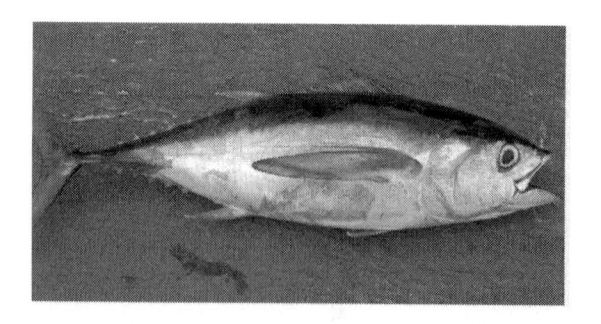

Tuna is a good source of protein, selenium, potassium, niacin, phosphorous, zinc, calcium, and vitamin B12.

1 can (165g) of drained light tuna contains, Calories: 191, Fat: 1.4g, Sodium: 83mg, Sugar: 0g, Protein: 42g.

5. Catfish

Catfish has a sweet, mild taste and is a good source of vitamins, nutrients, and minerals. Catfish is regularly seen worldwide on restaurant menus.

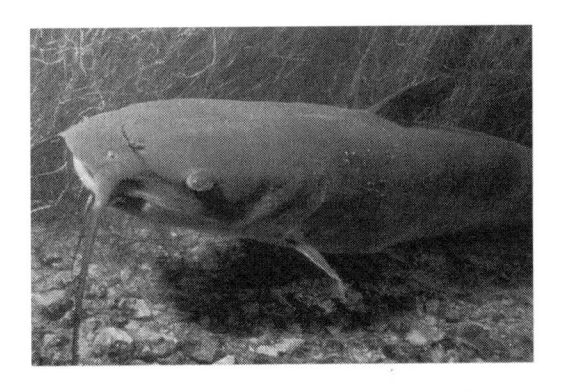

It is ZERO CARB food

Catfish is high protein seafood, vitamin B12, selenium, omega-3 and omega-6 fatty acids and has low calorie

Chapter Four

Shell food

List of shell food

Shellfish is one of the world's most nutritious foods, and people hardly noticed it.

It contains a LOW CARB of 4-5 % per 100 grams serving.

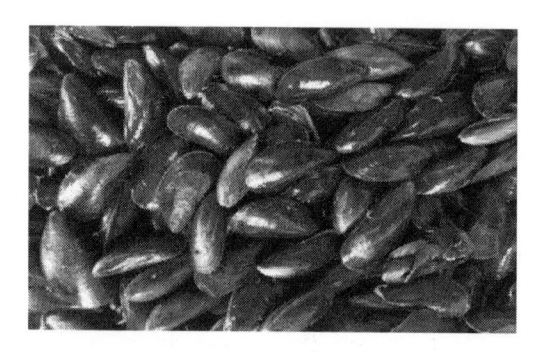

1. Shrimp

Shrimp is one of the world most nutritious foods and commonly consumed types of shellfish.

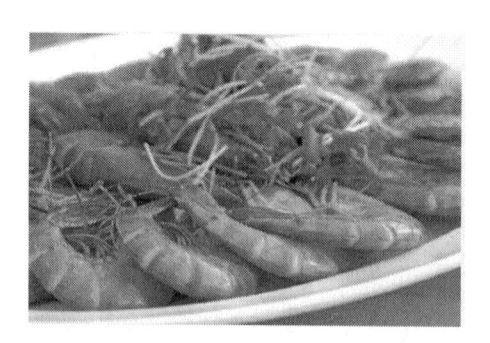

It contains ZERO CARB and rich in iodine, high in protein, and omega 3 and omega 6 fatty acids.

2. Haddock

Haddock fish is delicious and high nutritional food. It has a slightly sweet taste and delicate texture.

It contains ZERO CARB, high in protein, low mercury, no fiber, and no sugar

3. Lobster

Lobster meat is rich in healthy proteins. Lobsters are excellent source of selenium and also contain omega-3 fatty acids.

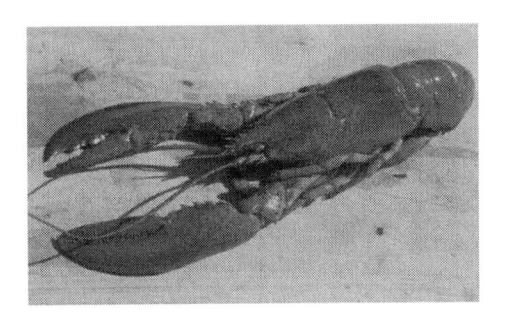

It contains ZERO CARB.

Lobster is a good source of zinc, Phosphorus, Vitamin B 12, Vitamin E, Magnesium, and Omega-3.

4. Herring

Herring is a nutritional and delicious type of oily fish.

It contains ZERO CARB, no fiber.

Herring fish is rich in vitamin A, vitamin B12, vitamin D, and folate. It is also a good source of calcium, magnesium, phosphorous, potassium, and omega 3 fatty acids.

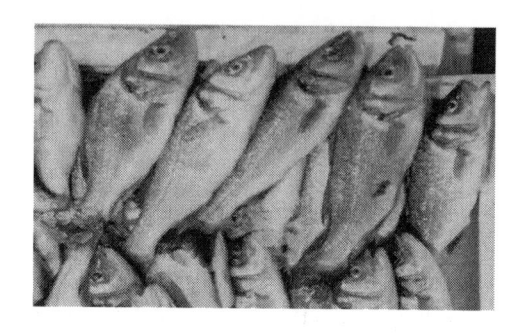

3 ounces of cooked herring contains 173 calories, 19.6g of protein, and 9.9g of fat.

Chapter Five

Vegetables

List of Vegetables

Many vegetables are low in carb and calories but high in vitamins, fiber, minerals, and other vital nutrients, making them perfect for low carb diets.

Vegetables that grow above the ground are generally low carb and can be eaten at will (be careful on quantity if you are on low carb diet).

Low carb diets vary for individuals. Most people opt for below 150 grams serving of carb per day while other do drastically down to 21 grams, serving of low-carb diets per day.

1. **Broccoli (4g)**

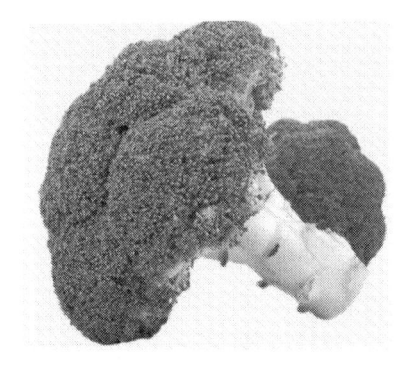

It is a LOW CARB (4g) veg.

Broccoli is a super tasty cruciferous vegetable.

It can be enjoyed cooked or raw. It's rich in vitamin C, vitamin K, and fiber.

Broccoli contains 4 grams Carb per 100 grams (3½ ounces) serving.

2. Tomatoes(4g)

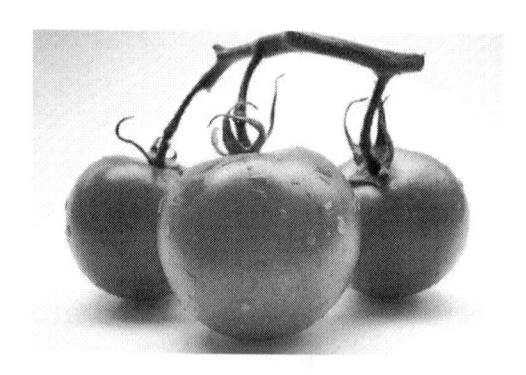

It is a LOW CARB (4g) veg

Tomatoes are classified as fruits but generally consumed as vegetables. Tomatoes are rich in potassium and vitamin C.

Tomatoes contain 4 grams of carb per 100 grams serving.

3. Brussels sprouts(5g)

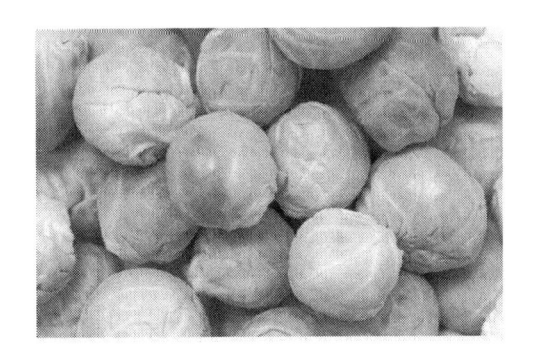

It a LOW CARB (5g) Veg

Brussels sprouts are tasty and highly nutritious vegetables. It contains a lot of beneficial compounds.

It is also a great source of vitamins K and C and antioxidants.

Brussels sprouts contain 5 grams of carb per 100 grams serving.

4. **Cauliflower (3g)**

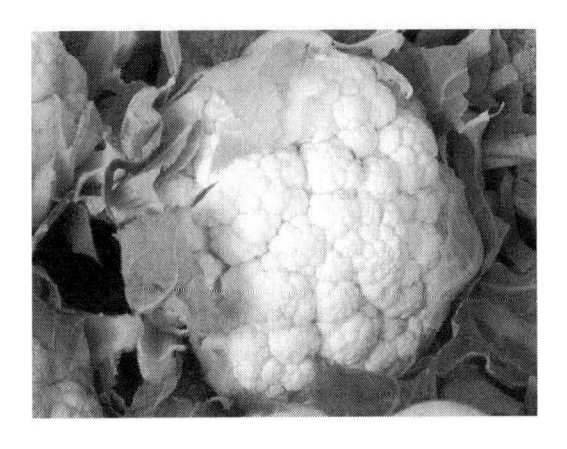

It is a LOW CARB (3g) Veg.

Cauliflower is the most classic and tasty low carb vegetable. It can be used to make a wide range of dishes in the kitchen. This versatile vegetable is high in folate, vitamin C and vitamin K

Cauliflowers contain 3 grams of carb per 100 grams servings.

5. Cabbage (3g)

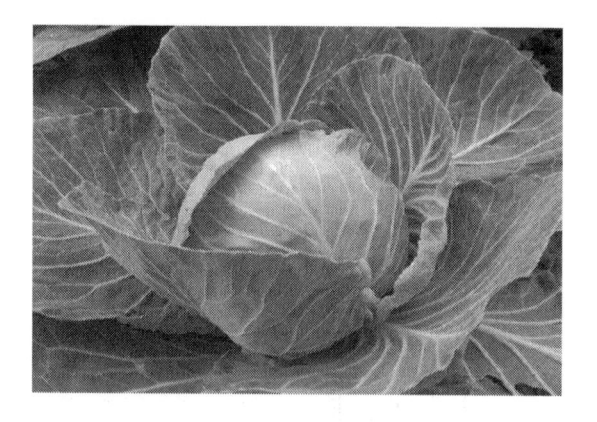

It is a LOW CARB (3g) Veg.

Cabbage is another tasty low-carb vegetable.

It is a cruciferous vegetable rich in vitamin C and K.

Cabbage contains 3 grams of carb per 100 grams serving.

6. Kale (3g)

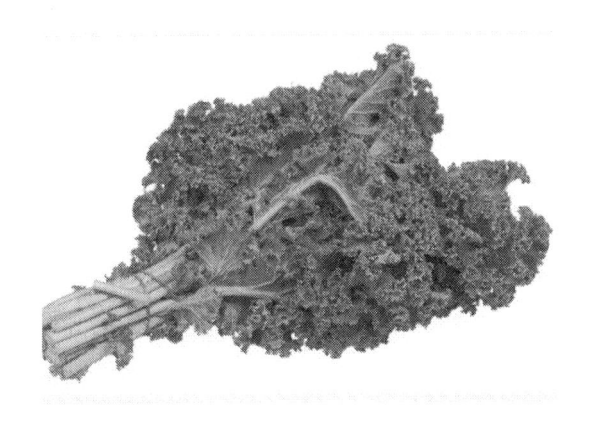

Kale is one of the most popular vegetables among people on low carb. It is less watery and harder when compared to spinach. Kale is enriched with numerous health benefits such as Vitamins C and K, Fiber, and Carotene antioxidants.

Cabbage contains 3 grams of carb per 100 grams serving.

7. **Eggplant (6g)**

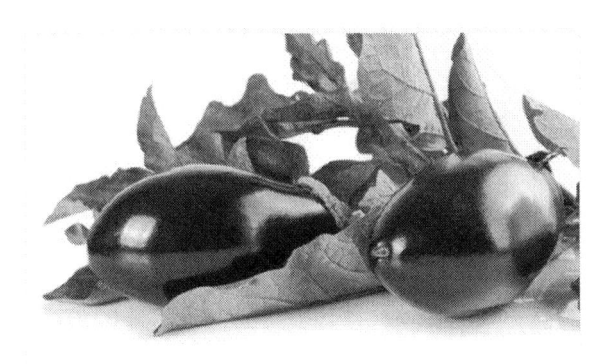

It is a LOW CARB (6g) Veg.

Eggplant is a fruit but widely eaten as a vegetable.

It offers a plentiful amount of vitamins, fiber, and minerals.

An eggplant contains 5 grams of carb per 100 grams serving.

8. Cucumber (4g)

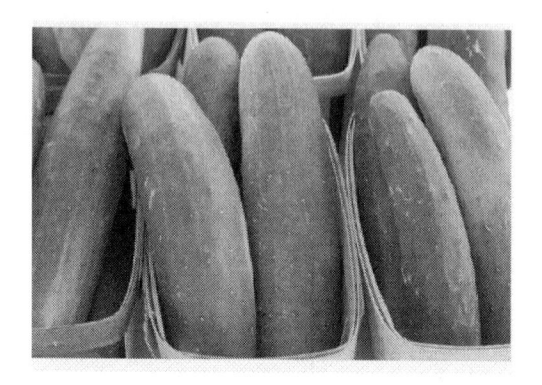

It is a LOW CARB (4g) Veg.

Cucumber is another vegetable that is widely consumed. It has a mild flavor and consists mostly of water. It contains Vitamin K in a small quantity.

Cucumbers contain 4 grams of carb per 100 grams serving.

9. Bell Peppers (6g)

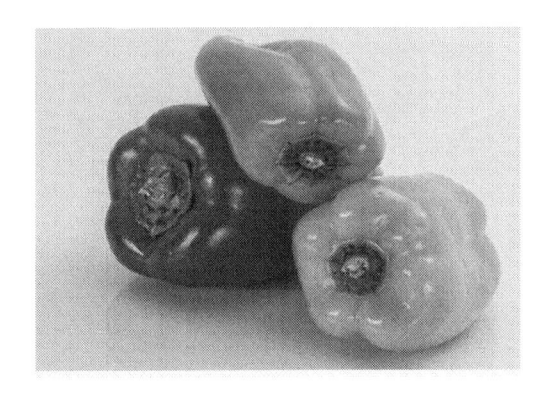

It is a LOW CARB (6g) Veg.

Fresh, raw bell peppers are popular vegetables with distinct taste and flavor. About 91.5% of its composition is water (92%) with a small quantity of fat, protein Vitamins, minerals, and carotene antioxidants.

Bell pepper contains 6 grams of carb per 100 grams serving.

10. Asparagus (2g)

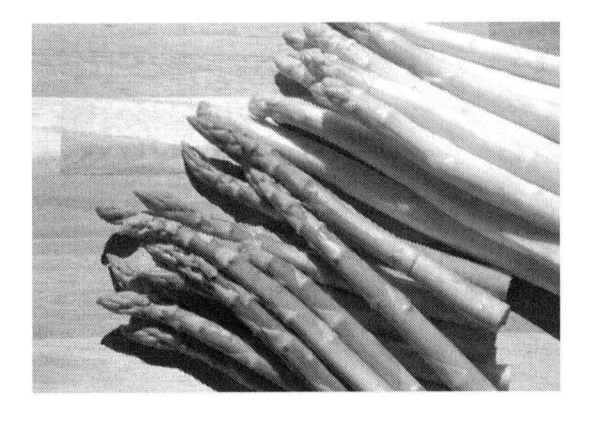

It is a LOW CARB (2g) Veg.

Asparagus is among the world's oldest cultivated vegetables. It is a highly tasty and nutritious spring vegetables. Asparagus is high in vitamin C and K, folate, fiber, and carotene antioxidants. It is an excellent source of protein when compared to most vegetables

Asparagus contains 2 grams of carb per 100 grams serving.

11. Green Beans (4g)

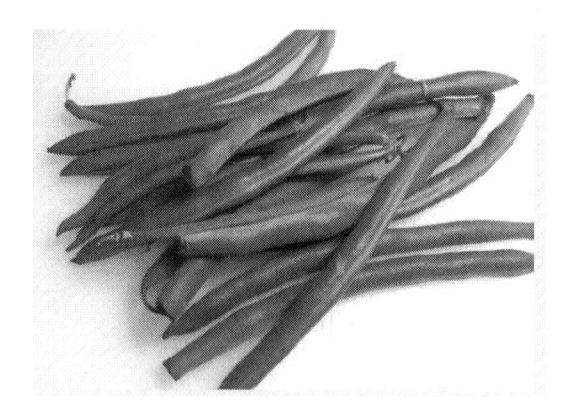

It is a LOW CARB (4g) Veg.

Green beans are tasty and delicious vegetables that can also be classified as legumes. Green beans taste great when cooked with butter or bacon

They are an excellent source of nutrients in high proportions. The nutrients are fiber, Vitamin C and K, protein, magnesium, and potassium.

Green beans contain 4 grams of carb per 100 grams serving.

12. Mushrooms (3g)

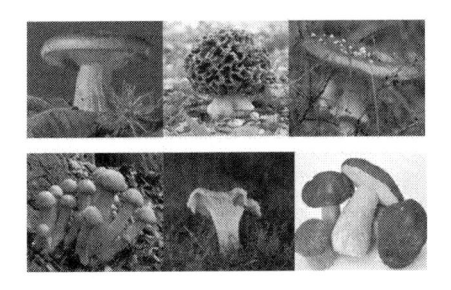

It is a LOW CARB (3g) Veg.

Edible mushrooms are groups as vegetables. Mushrooms are not only tasty but highly nutritious as well. They are packed with vitamins and minerals such as B vitamins and potassium.

Mushrooms (white) contain 3 grams of carb per 100 grams serving.

13. Spinach (1g)

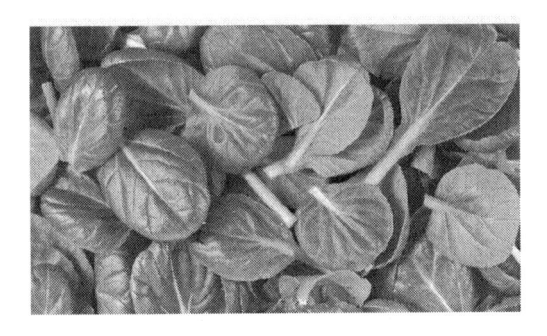

It is a LOW CARB (1%) Veg.

Spinach is an extremely low-carb vegetable. Spinach is very tasty when used with eggs. It is loaded with vitamins and minerals.

Spinach contains 1 gram of carb per 100 grams serving.

14. Zucchini (3 g)

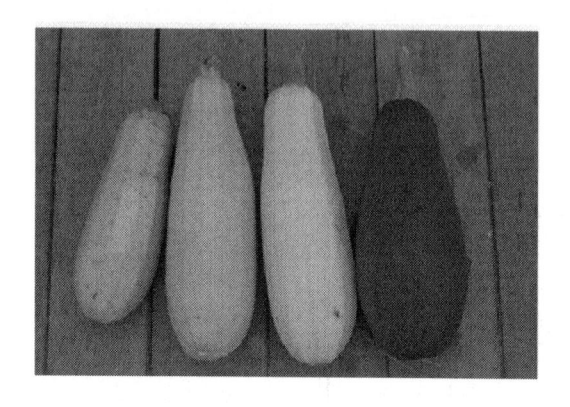

It is a LOW CARB (3g) Veg.

Zucchini is a super low carb vegetable. It is also classified as a fruit. Zucchini is enriched with varieties of minerals, vitamins, and other essential plant compounds. When cooked, the vitamin contents in zucchini increases.

Zucchini contains 3 grams of carb per 100 grams serving.

15. Celery (3g)

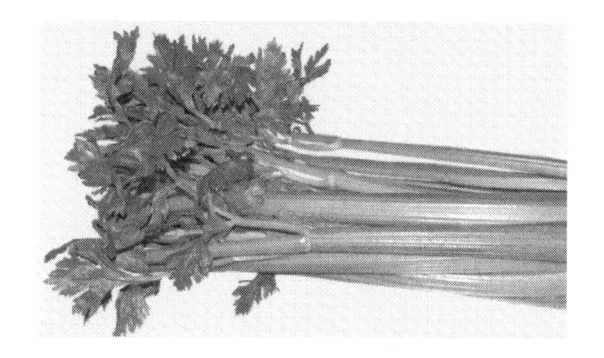

It is a LOW CARB (3g) Veg.

Celery is a green leaf vegetable with a distinct flavor and great taste. It is high in antioxidants, Vitamin C. flavonoids, and beta carotene. 95 % content of celery is water; the rest is soluble and insoluble fiber.

Celery contains 3 grams of carb per 100 grams serving.

16. Swiss chard (4g)

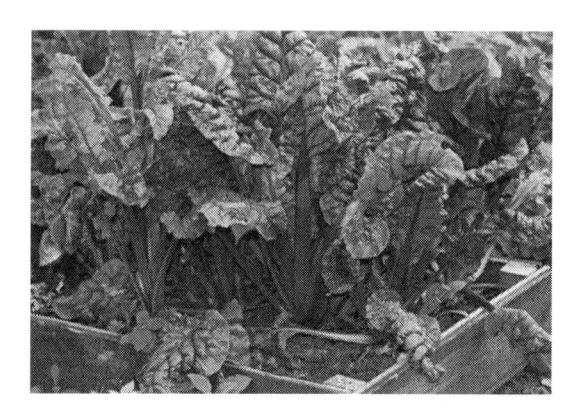

It is a LOW CARB (4g) Veg.

Swiss chard is one of the most nutrient-dense green vegetables with a dark, leafy body. This delicious vegetable is consumed all over the world.

Swiss chard has a lot of nutritional benefits.

Swiss chard contains 4 grams of carb per 100 grams serving.

17. Avocado (2 g).

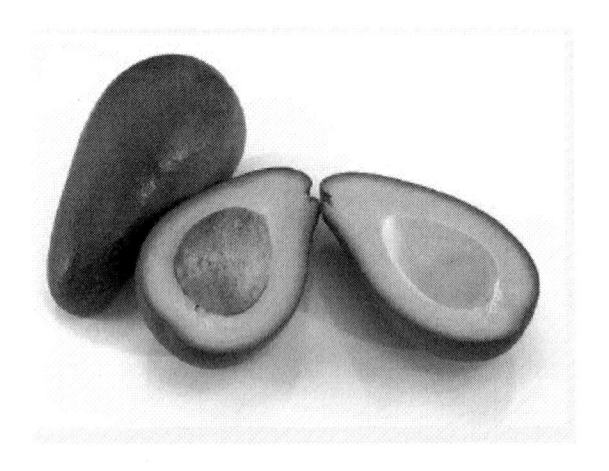

It is a LOW CARB (2g) Veg.

Avocado is a unique type of fruit but is graded as a vegetable. It is low in carb, extremely high in fiber, and loaded with nutritious fat. It also contains potassium and a decent amount of other nutrients.

Avocado contains 2 grams of carbs per 100 grams serving.

Chapter Six

Fruits and berries

Lists of fruits and berries

The best fruits and berries to eat on a low-carb diet are listed below. Most fruits and berries are okay when they are eaten in moderation for those on a low carb diet. Some people who eat fruits as candy should know that fruit contains a lot of sugar, and it might not be suitable for you in a large proportion if you are following a low carb diet.

If you are on a low diet, the amount of fruit you take depends on the quantity of carb you want to consume per day. It is recommended to restrict the amount of fruit you take to 1 per day.

It is not a good idea for a person who is on a low carb diet of 20 grams per day to eat fruit. You can get all the ingredients you need in a day from vegetables. Another option you can substitute for fruits is a berry, yes berry is fairly okay.

1. **Olives (6g)**

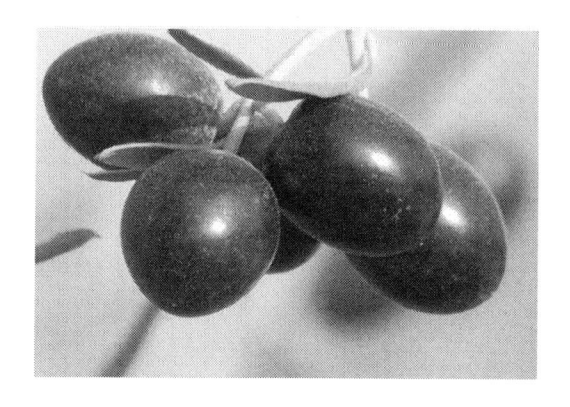

It is a LOW CARB (6g) fruit.

They have a rich, salty taste and a chewy texture.

The olive is delicious high-fat fruit with a rich, salty taste. Olive is rich in copper, iron and contains a moderate amount of vitamin E.

Olive contains 6 grams of carb per 100 grams serving.

2. Strawberries (6g)

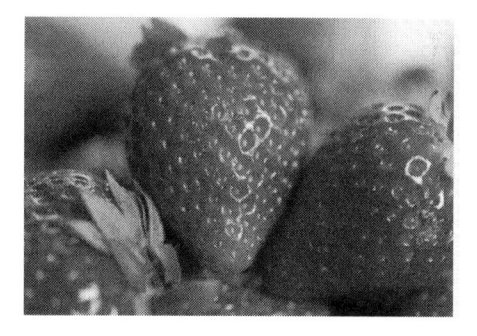

It is a LOW CARB (6g) fruit.

Strawberries are graded as one of the lowest-carb and most nutrient-dense fruits you can consume while on a low carb diet. Strawberries are rich in manganese, vitamin C, and a lot of antioxidants.

Strawberries contain 6 grams of carb per 100 grams serving.

3. Grapefruit (11g)

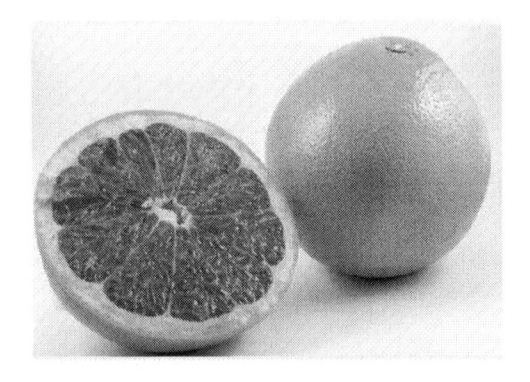

It is a LOW CARB (11g) fruit.

Grapefruit is a citrus fruit with bittersweet to sour flavor. It is related to oranges and is high vitamins and minerals. Grapefruits enriched vitamin C and carotene antioxidants.

Grapefruits contain 11 grams of carb per 100 grams serving.

4. Apricots (11g)

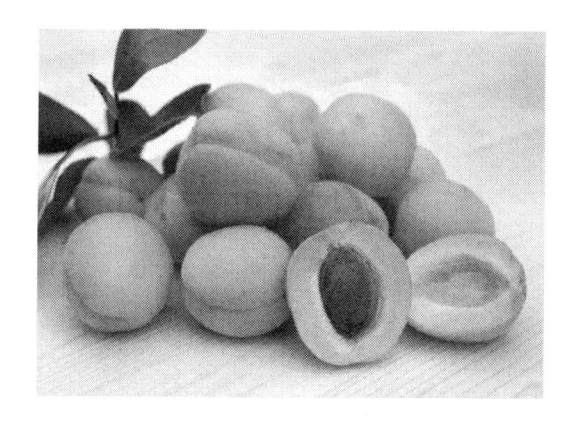

It is a LOW CARB (11g) fruit.

Apricots are incredibly delicious stone fruits. They are incredibly nutritious fruit and have a lot of vitamin C and potassium.

Apricots contain 11 grams of carb per 100 grams serving.

5. Raspberries (5g)

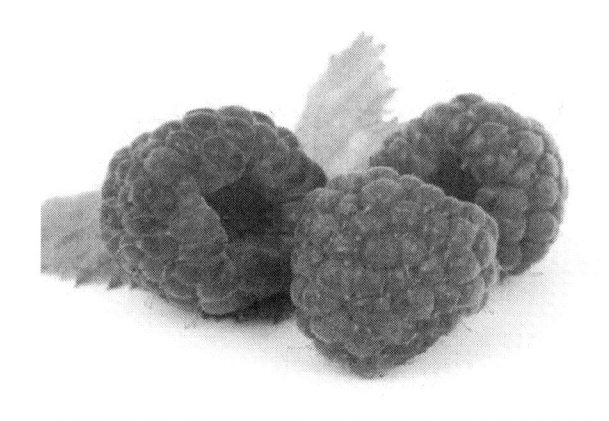

It is a LOW CARB (5g) fruit.

Raspberries are sweet edible fruit in the rose family packed with essential vitamins and minerals like vitamin C and fiber.

Raspberries contain 5 grams of carb per 100 grams serving.

6. Blackberries (6.5 g)

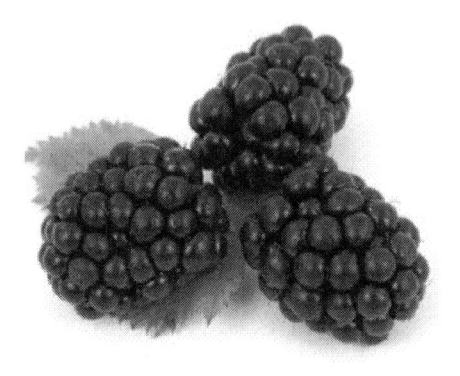

It is a LOW CARB (6.5g) fruit.

Blackberries are delicious berries that can be added to any diet. They are also packed with vital antioxidants and nutrients. Blackberries are a great source of manganese, vitamin C, and fiber.

Blackberries contain 6.5 grams of carb per 100 grams serving.

7. Kiwis (12g)

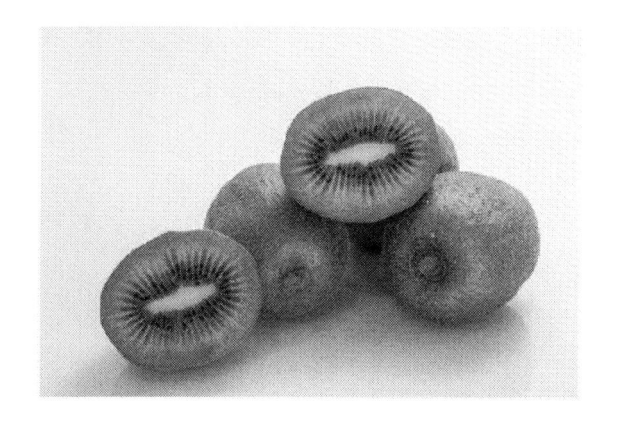

It is a LOW CARB (12g) fruit.

Kiwis are small delicious fruits with sweet and tangy flavor. It's a great source of vitamin C, K, and E, folate, and potassium. A good source of fiber and rich with many antioxidants.

Kiwis contain 12 grams of carb per 100 grams serving.

8. Lemons(6g)

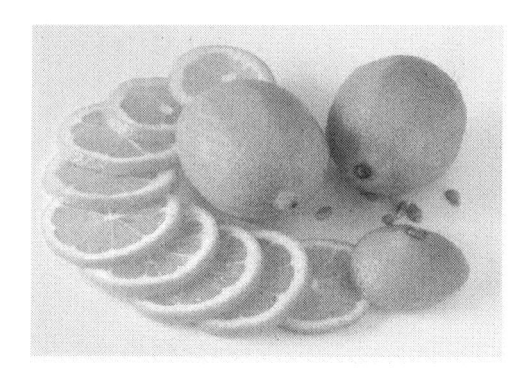

It is a LOW CARB (6g) fruit.

Lemons are among the citrus fruit that are widely consumed. Lemons have a sour taste and are full of vitamins, phytonutrients, minerals, fiber, folate and antioxidants.

Lemons contain 9.3 grams of carb per 100 grams serving.

Chapter Seven

Nuts and seeds

Lists of Nuts and Seeds

Nuts are dry, single-seeded fruits with high oil content, bounded in a sturdy outer cover. Nuts and seeds are known to be essential energy and nutrients sources all over the world.

They are a reliable and delicious source of essential nutrients and very popular among people on a low carb diet. Nuts and seeds are high in fiber, low in carbs, fat, protein, and many micronutrients. Most people eat nuts and seeds as snacks, crunch to salads or recipes.

People on a low carb diet are to eat one serving of nuts and seeds per day.

NOTE

100 grams = about 3 handfuls.

1. **Almonds (9 g)**

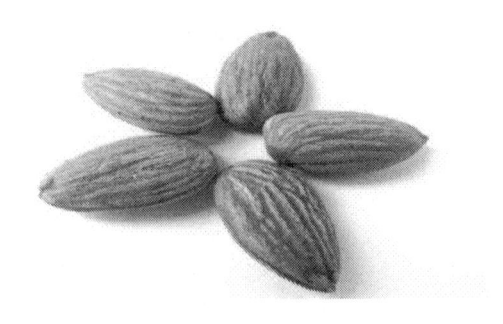

It is a LOW CARB (9g) nut.

Almonds are an incredibly crunchy and tasty nut. Almonds are among the most popular nuts in the United States.

They are packed with vitamin E, fiber, and magnesium.

Almonds contain 9 grams of carb per 100 grams serving.

2. Walnuts (7g)

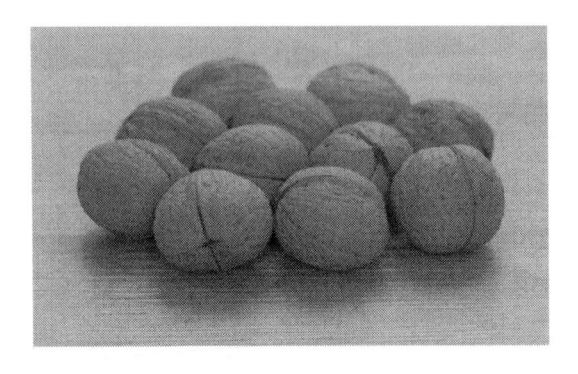

It is a LOW CARB (7g) nut.

Walnuts are round; single delicious seeded stone nuts that grow from the walnut tree. They are abundant in healthful fats, fiber, and protein. Walnuts are exceptionally high in omega-3 fatty acids.

Walnuts contain 7 grams of carb per 100 grams serving.

3. Peanuts (8g)

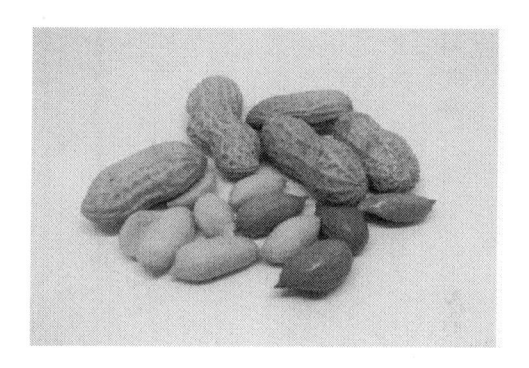

It is a LOW CARB (8g) nut.

Peanuts are crunchy, delicious nutty oilseeds known to people since centuries ago.

Peanuts are abundant in plant-based protein, fiber, fat, Vitamin E, and magnesium.

Peanuts contain 8 grams of carb per 100 grams serving.

4. Pecan (7g)

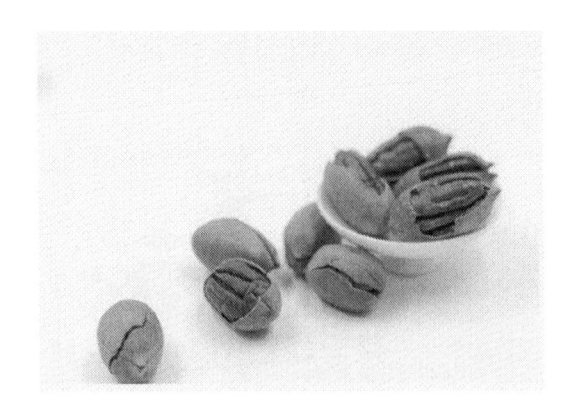

It is a LOW CARB (7g) nut.

The pecans are delicious, crunchy, and healthy nuts with contoured structure. Its buttery flavor makes for exciting ingredients to contain in several dishes.

Pecans contain 7 grams of carb per 100 grams serving.

5. Brazil (4g)

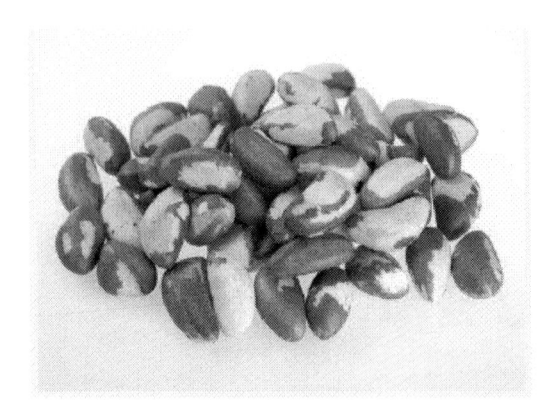

It is a LOW CARB (4g) nut.

Brazil is delicious and very unique nuts. Brazil nuts are packed with many powerful nutritional benefits. They are a great source of protein and contain a lot of amino acids.

Brazil nuts contain 4 grams of carb per 100 grams serving.

6. Macadamia (5g)

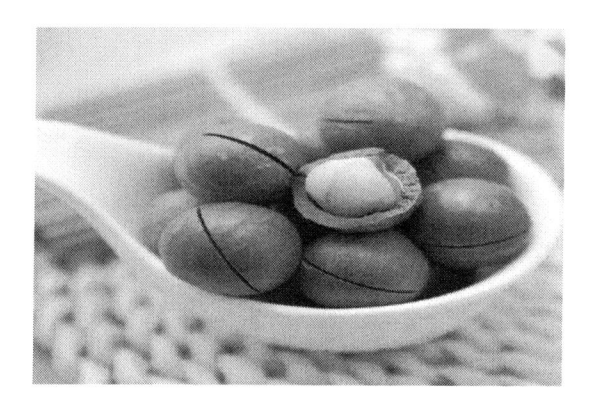

It is a LOW CARB (5g) nut.

Macadamia nuts are delicious with a creamy texture and butter-like flavor. They are high in healthy fats, contains dietary fiber, manganese, protein, and copper.

Macadamia nuts contain 5 grams of carb per 100 grams serving.

7. Pine (9g)

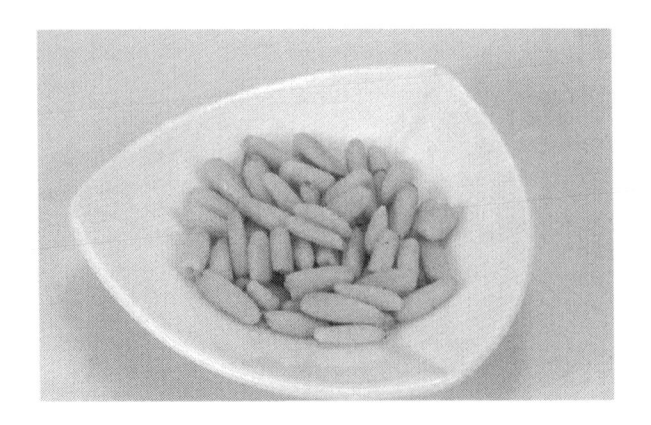

It is a LOW CARB (9g) nut.

Pine nuts are seed collected from some types of pine cones. These nuts are delicious, crunchy, and tasty with a buttery flavor. Pine is enriched with healthy fats

Pine nuts contain 5 grams of carb per 100 grams serving.

8. Hazelnuts (7g)

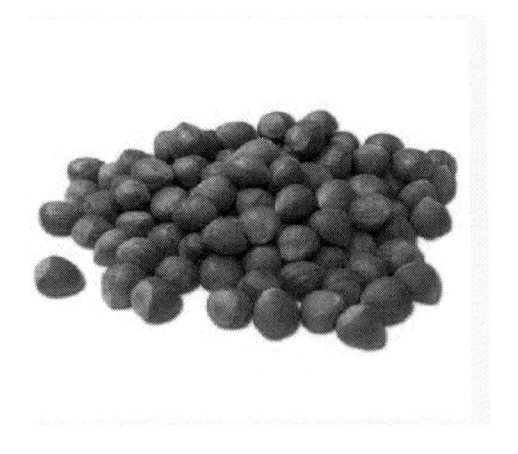

It is a LOW CARB (7g) nut.

Hazelnuts are among the popular delicious nut that can be eaten roasted, raw or ground into a paste. They have a sweet flavor and are rich in nutrients. Hazelnuts are abundant in healthful, fats, protein, vitamins, dietary fiber, and minerals.

Hazelnuts contain 7 grams of carb per 100 grams serving.

9. Coconut (6g)

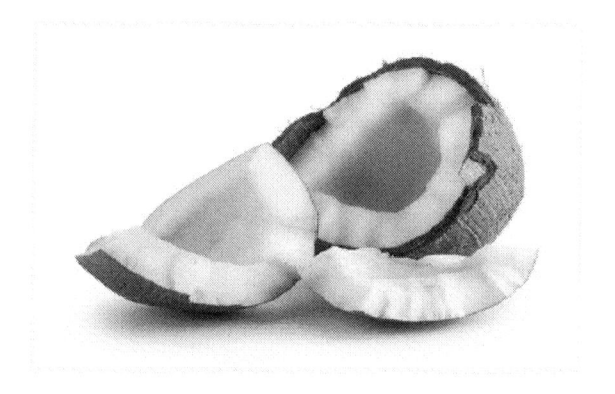

It is a LOW CARB (6g) nut.

Coconut meat is white and tasty with a firm texture. The meat has a slightly sweet flavor. Coconut meat can be eaten raw or dried.

Coconut meat is mainly high in fibers, calories, and saturated fat. It's also a source of manganese, selenium, copper, phosphorus, iron, and potassium.

Coconut contains 6 grams of carb per 100 grams serving.

10. Flaxseeds (28 g)

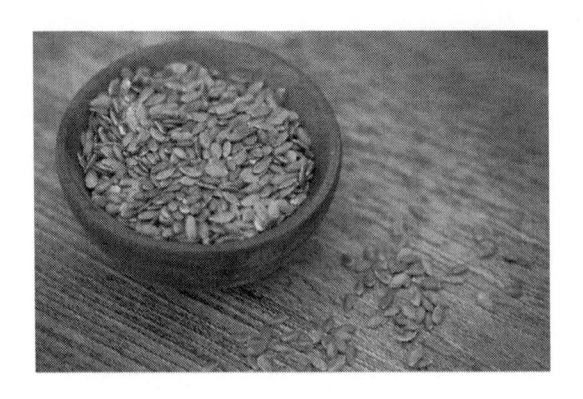

It is a LOW CARB (28g) nut.

Flaxseeds are among the most potent plant food in the universe. They provide the body with an extraordinary amount of healthful fat, fiber and antioxidants, protein, and omega-3 fatty acids.

A typical serving =1 tablespoon = 7 grams. = 2 grams carb.

Flaxseeds contain 28 grams of carb per 100 grams serving.

11. Pumpkin seeds (15 g)

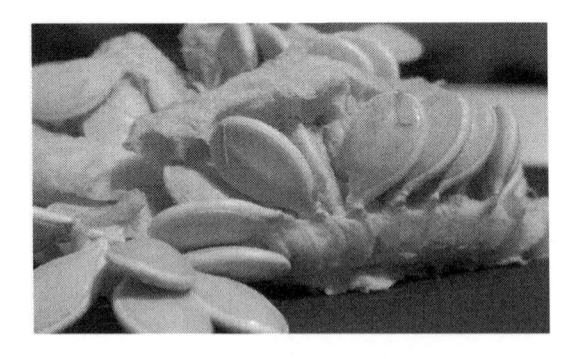

It is a LOW CARB (15g) nut.

Pumpkin seeds are edible, delicious seeds that are roasted before consumption. They are a great source of antioxidants, zinc, iron, magnesium, plant protein and a lot of nutrients

Pumpkin seeds contain 15 grams of carb per 100 grams serving.

12. Sunflower seeds (21g).

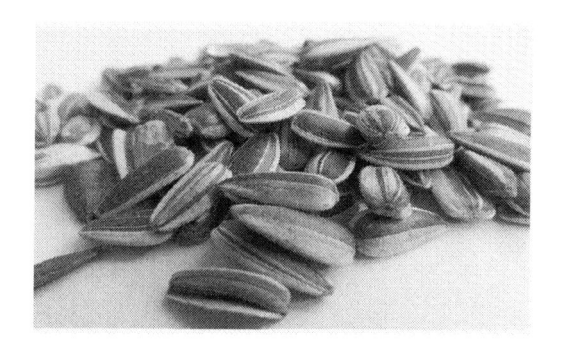

It is a LOW CARB (21g) nut.

Sunflower seeds are tasty, rich seeds that many choose to ignore. They are high in healthy fats, a great source of protein, fats, minerals, vitamins, and beneficial plant compounds.

Sunflower contains 21 grams of carb per 100 grams serving.

Chapter Eight

Dairy

List of dairy

Full-fat dairy is a great low–carb food for people that can put up with dairy. It makes a great list for a low carb keto list. Dairy foods are delicious, and they give vital nutrients to the body. Before you purchase any full-fat dairy product, check and read the nutrition label at the back to avoid buying anything with added sugar.

1. **Butter (0 g)**

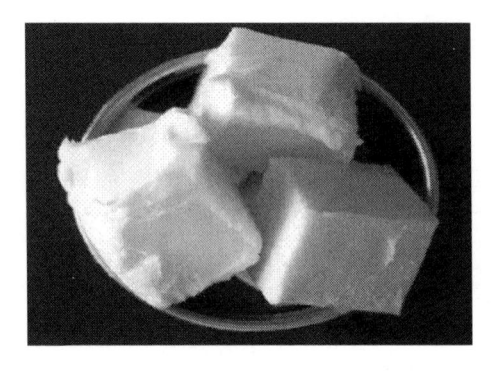

It is a LOW CARB (0g) dairy.

Butter is a known dairy product prepared from cow's milk by churning the cream to remove the extra liquid.

It has a great flavor and is generally used as a spread for baking and cooking. Butter is high in calories and fat.

Butter has no carb, no fiber making it a low glycemic, low carb food.

Butter contains 0 grams of carb per 100 grams serving.

2. Cream Cheese (4g)

It is a LOW CARB (4g) dairy.

Cream cheese is soft, has a smooth consistency, and one of the tastiest low carb foods. It is a typical spread for bread, bagels, and crackers. Cheese is high in nutrients and a great source of vitamin A, little of riboflavin (Vitamin B2). It also rich in fat and contains a small number of carbs and protein.

Cream Cheese contains 4 grams of carb per 100 grams serving.

3. Heavy Cream (3g)

It is a LOW CARB (3g) dairy.

Heavy cream is delicious when added to a meal, for example, in a coffee or a bowl of berries.

Heavy cream is high in dairy fat, but contains very few carbs and little protein.

Heavy cream contains 3 grams of carb per 100 grams serving.

4. Mayonnaise (1g)

It is a LOW CARB (1g) dairy.

Mayonnaise makes a delicious meal when used in sandwiches, dressings, and salads. It is packed with various minerals and vitamins. Mayonnaise is abundant in vitamin E, vitamin K and high in fats and calories but low in fiber and protein.

Mayonnaise contains 1 gram of carb per 100 grams serving.

5. Full-fat yogurt (5g)

It is a LOW CARB (5g) dairy.

Yogurt is among the common fermented dairy product that is consumed widely. Yogurt is loaded with useful probiotic bacteria.

Yogurt is abundant in high-quality protein, fats, and it contains small amounts of lactose. Beware of a brand that contains sugar and flavoring.

Full-fat yoghurt contains 5 grams of carb per 100 grams serving.

6. Greek Yogurt (4g)

It is a LOW CARB (4g) dairy

Greek yogurt is a common dairy product that is consumed widely.

The difference between Greek yogurt and other yogurt is that Greek yogurt does not have whey. "Whey" is a liquid that contains lactose and natural sugar presence in milk. Greek yogurt is abundant in many useful nutrients such as calcium, protein, probiotics, iodine, and vitamin B-12.

Greek yogurt contains 4 grams of carb per 100 grams serving.

7. Béarnaise (2g)

It is a LOW CARB (2g) dairy.

A béarnaise sauce is delicious tasty low- carb foods designed especially for people on a low carb diet. It comprises egg yolk, white wine vinegar, onion powder, fresh chopped tarragon, butter, salt, and pepper. Béarnaise sauce is packed with vital minerals and vitamins.

Béarnaise contains 2 grams of carb per 100 grams serving.

8. Salsa (6g)

Salsa is a common condiment that is used all over the world. Fresh salsa adds distinct flavor and nutrients to food.

9. Other low-carb dairies are:
- Aioli (2g)
- Soy Sauce (4 g)
- Guacamole (3g)

- Vinaigrette (3 g)

Vinaigrette is a healthy salad dressing for people on a low carb diet.

- Mustard (6g)
- Pesto (8 g)

Chapter Nine

Fats and Oils

Lists of fats and oils

There are a lot of healthy fats and oils that are suitable for low-carb.

1. Butter (Zero)

It is a ZERO CARB (0g) fat

Butter is a great source of fat for cooking and frying. Choose grass-fed butter if possible because of its high nutritional value.

2. Extra Virgin Olive Oil (Zero)

It is ZERO CARB (0g) oil

Extra virgin olive oil is an exceptional healthy oil and among the best edible oils in the world. The oil is endowed with a pleasant flavor, antioxidant properties, and numerous health benefits.

3. Coconut Oil (Zero)

It is ZERO CARB (0g) oil

Coconut oil is also an exceptional healthy fat, loaded with a medium-chain fatty acid, and vitamin E. Coconut oil also contains no fiber and little minerals.

4. Avocado oil (Zero)

It is ZERO CARB (0g) oil

Avocado oil is delicious oil extracted from avocado fruit. It's high in healthy fats and antioxidants. Oleic oil is the most abundant fatty acids in avocado oil, and it offers many health benefits.

5. Lard (zero)

It is ZERO CARB (0g) fat

Lard is another very versatile fat, and fats present in lard are good fats, which is called monounsaturated fats. They are an excellent option for deep frying, frying and baking.

6. Tallow (zero)

Tallow is a fat extracted for beef and is suitable for frying, baking, and cooking. Tallow is a good source of Vitamins A, D, E, and K

Chapter Ten

Beverages

Sugar-free beverages are great on a low-carb diet. Water is a perfect example of a low carb beverage. Keeping yourself well hydrated is vital to feeling good. There are lots of low carb alcoholic and non-alcoholic beverages you can enjoy while on low-carb food.

Fruit juice is not advisable for those on a low carb diet because it contains a lot of sugar and also high in carb.

You can still enjoy low-carb alcoholic beverages in moderation while on a low carb diet.

Some pure alcohol products like rum, gin, vodka, tequila and whiskey contain no carbs but wine and light beer fairly low in carbs.

1. **Water (Zero)**

Water is still the best beverage to take on low-carb. Drinking water regularly while on a low carb diet can reduce headaches, fatigue, dry mouth, and flu-like symptoms caused by dehydration. This dehydration is a result of a decrease in carbohydrates intake.

2. **Coffee (Zero)**

Coffee is one of the most common beverages consumed all over the world. Coffee has a delicious fragrance, intense flavor, and caffeine, and an excellent source of dietary antioxidants.

Avoid adding unhealthy things to your coffee. Keep it simple and black or you can add some heavy cream or full-fat milk.

3. Tea (Zero)

Not just tea but green tea. Green tea is widely known as a healthy drink, packed with many exciting health benefits.

4. Club Soda / Carbonated Water (Zero)

Club soda is when carbon dioxide and water are mixed together. It is also a perfect drink for low carb diet. Drink only the sugar free one. Ensure you read the label before purchasing.

Other Food

They are also some food suitable for low carb diet.

1. Dark Chocolate (LOW)

Real dark chocolate with a minimum of 70-85% cocoa is a perfect low carb treat.

It comes with its health benefits.

2. Herbs, Spices, and Condiments

There are varieties of tasty herbs, condiments and spices. Majorities are very low in carbs but full powerful nutritional punch and add flavor to meals.

Printed in Great Britain
by Amazon